DIY Natural Beauty Products

Glowing Skin Delights

Hina Victor

Dedication

This devotion is for you - the ones who accept that excellence can be both regular and practical, without settling on viability. For the visionaries embrace the effortlessness and sorcery of nature, looking for excellence for the outside appearance as well as for the prosperity of their bodies and the planet.

In this speedy world, we frequently wind up barraged with business magnificence items loaded up with synthetics and engineered fixings, promising handy solutions and short-term changes. In any case, in this quest for magnificence, we may be accidentally hurting our bodies and adding to the debasement of our current circumstance.

This devotion is an update that we have the ability to assume control over issues. We can decide to set out on an excursion of taking care of oneself, magnificence, and manageability by making our own regular excellence items.

To the people who have previously started this excursion, I praise your devotion to bettering yourself and the planet. You are the trailblazers of a development that encourages a significant association with nature, understanding that the World's assets can give all the sustenance and care we really want.

To the people who are simply beginning, realize that you are in good company. Embracing the Do-It-Yourself way might appear to be overwhelming from the outset, however with a touch of information, imagination, and persistence, you will reveal a universe of vast conceivable outcomes and advantages that locally acquired items can't recreate.

Making your regular excellence items permits you to fit details to suit your special skin type and inclinations. It engages you to choose morally obtained, savagery free, and eco-accommodating fixings that regard every living being and the planet we share.

By committing yourself to Do-It-Yourself regular excellence items, you embrace the craft of confidence and self-articulation. You find that genuine excellence emanates from the inside and that the ceremonies of blending, mixing, and spoiling can be both helpful and enabling.

This commitment reaches out to Earth's life giving force herself. By picking regular fixings and lessening our dependence on unsafe synthetic substances, we assume a little yet critical part in protecting the world's fragile equilibrium. We can diminish plastic waste, limit the contamination brought about by business magnificence ventures, and add to a cleaner, greener planet for a long time into the future.

In this excursion, you might experience difficulties and misfortunes, yet recall that each step you make is a stride towards a better and more agreeable way of life. Embrace the educational experience, share your revelations with others, and motivate people around you to embrace the magnificence of nature.

To all who trust in the groundbreaking force of regular excellence items and the magnificence of changing our reality to improve things, this devotion is for you. Allow us to proceed with this way together, with affection, commitment, and a common vision for an additional economical and lovely future.

Hina Victor

Table of Contents

Foreword

Welcome to the charming universe of Do-It-Yourself normal magnificence items. Inside these pages, you will leave on an excursion that commends the excellence of nature and the craft of taking care of oneself. As you dig into the domains of blending, mixing, and making your excellence creations, you will find the gigantic power that lies in your grasp - the ability to change your actual appearance, however your whole way to deal with magnificence and prosperity.

In a world immersed with business excellence items, overflowing with counterfeit fixings and commitments of supernatural occurrences, neglecting to focus on the genuine pith of beauty is simple. This foreword fills in as a delicate update that external appeal isn't simply superficial; it radiates from the inside, joined with the embroidery of nature's marvels.

The Do-It-Yourself normal magnificence development is certainly not a simple pattern; it is a way of thinking established together as one and supportability. By selecting to create your excellence items, you are pursuing a cognizant choice to respect your body and the climate. You move back from the ocean of efficiently manufactured things, each conveying a weighty natural impression, and embrace a way that prompts a greener, more humane presence.

This book is your compass, directing you through the tremendous scene of normal fixings, excellence customs, and helpful cures. You will figure out how to saddle the integrity of botanicals, natural ointments, and supporting concentrates that have been treasured for a really long time by our precursors.

In any case, past the useful skill, this excursion will light your imagination. Trial and error will turn into your dream, as need might arise and inclinations. There are no limits, just the immense material of nature sitting tight for you to investigate and paint your magnificence magnum opus.

However, with this artistic liberty comes liability. As you draw in with nature's gifts, you'll acquire a freshly discovered appreciation for its delicacy. This mindfulness will fuel your devotion to protecting the world's assets and regarding all living things. Each time you blend an elixir or apply an ointment, you'll do as such with a careful heart, realizing that your decisions swell past yourself.

I commend your boldness in following the way more uncommon, for it is through your interest and responsibility that the world will embrace a more economical future. Embrace the educational experience, for there is excellence in each mix-up and development in each victory.

May this book be your steady friend, rousing you to implant love and aim into each hand tailored creation. Allow it to be a demonstration of the significant association between people and the regular world, a bond that should be sustained and secured.

As you set out on this experience, recollect that magnificence isn't tied in with accomplishing impossible norms, yet about praising the uniqueness of what your identity is. It's tied in with treasuring the magnificence of your general surroundings and being aware of your decisions.

With open hearts and receptive outlooks, let us set out together on this groundbreaking excursion of Do-It-Yourself regular excellence. May it lead us to a position of legitimacy, where we rediscover the brilliance of our spirits and the brightness o f the planet we call home

Hina Victor

Preface

In a world loaded up with a consistently developing cluster of magnificence items, each encouraging to be a wonder in a container, it is not difficult to become overpowered and detached from the genuine quintessence of taking care of oneself. As we are besieged with ostentatious ads and captivating promoting methodologies, we might wind up looking for handy solutions and moment changes, frequently at the expense of our wellbeing and the climate.

This introduction fills in as a genuine greeting to move away from the turbulent universe of business magnificence and embrace the effortlessness and virtue of Do-It-Yourself normal excellence items. In this excursion, we will uncover the mysteries of the Earth, saddling the plentiful gifts nature has gave to us, and changing them into supporting elixirs for the body, psyche, and soul.

The way of thinking of making our excellence items goes past the charm of setting aside cash or having a great time side interest. It is a careful decision to embrace a more cognizant way of life - one that is personally associated with the normal world. By creating our definitions, we gain a more profound comprehension of the fixings we use, their starting points, and their significant effect on our prosperity and the climate.

In the sections that follow, you will leave on a journey of disclosure. You will find out about the miracles of medicinal balms, the reviving properties of botanicals, and the recuperating capability of different spices and concentrates. Together, we will investigate the craft of mixing these components to make customized excellence cures, custom-made to suit your interesting skin type, hair surface, and individual inclinations.

The excellence of this excursion lies not just in the eventual outcomes that elegance your vanity however in the extraordinary cycle itself. As you submerge yourself in the realm of normal excellence, you will end up associating with the insight of previous eras, who worshipped the world's contributions to improve their magnificence and prosperity.

All through this book, I urge you to embrace your imagination, for the universe of Do-It-Yourself magnificence is unlimited. From making calming medicine to strengthening scours, and from feeding hair veils to fragrant shower mixes, the conceivable outcomes are restricted exclusively by your creative mind.

Yet, while we revel in the delight of imagination, we should likewise be aware of the obligation that accompanies it. As gatekeepers of the earth, it is our obligation to proceed with caution and morally. This excursion will motivate you to search out feasible, morally obtained, and remorselessness free fixings, adding to the general benefit of every residing being and the planet we call home.

I trust this prelude establishes the vibe for a charming and edifying experience. May you embrace this way with an open heart and a receptive outlook, permitting the excellence of nature to support you from the back to front.

As you leave on this journey of Do-It-Yourself normal excellence items, recall that taking care of oneself isn't an extravagance yet a need, and genuine magnificence is an impression of the adoration we develop for us and our general surroundings.

With limitless inventiveness and profound veneration for nature, let us set out together on this wondrous excursion of Do-It-Yourself normal magnificence items.

Hina Victor

Introduction

Welcome to the charming universe of Do-It-Yourself regular magnificence items! In this period of present day comforts and high speed ways of life, it's not difficult to fail to remember the ageless insight our predecessors had about bridling the force of nature for excellence and prosperity. This acquaintance fills in as your passage with rediscovering the craft of making customized, regular magnificence cures that support both your body and soul.

In our current reality where synthetic loaded excellence items rule the racks, the charm of Do-It-Yourself normal magnificence allures us with commitments of virtue, viability, and manageability. A development celebrates effortlessness, engaging people to assume command over their magnificence ceremonies and embrace the decency nature brings to the table.

The motivation behind this guide is to move you to investigate the huge mother lode of botanicals, spices, rejuvenating balms, and normal fixings that can change your taking care of oneself daily schedule into a custom of self esteem. Whether you are a carefully prepared Do-It-Yourself lover or an inquisitive beginner, there is something enchanted looking for you in these pages.

All through this excursion, you will find the endless advantages of picking normal elements for your magnificence needs. In addition to the fact that these components delicate on are your skin, hair, and by and large wellbeing, however they likewise accompany the additional benefit of being harmless to the ecosystem. By moving away from items containing unsafe synthetic substances and impractical assets, you are making a little however huge stride towards a greener, more caring world.

The magnificence of Do-It-Yourself normal excellence items lies in their viability as well as in the craft of creation itself. As you explore different avenues regarding various recipes and plans, you will track down happiness in mixing aromas, surfaces, and varieties. Every creation will be an impression of your interesting inclinations and necessities, making your excellence schedule a profoundly private and satisfying experience.

Whether you want to create a liberal spa-like insight, address explicit skin concerns, or just hug a more regular lifestyle, you will track down a heap of recipes, tips, and procedures inside these pages to direct you on your way.

Notwithstanding, it is crucial for approach this excursion with a receptive outlook and an eagerness to learn. Making regular excellence items is a workmanship, and like any art, it requires investment, practice, and persistence. Be encouraged by any setbacks or not exactly wonderful endeavors; rather, consider them to be potential chances to develop and refine your abilities.

Moreover, as you dive into this universe of normal fixings, recall the meaning of moral obtaining and supportability. Valuing the World's assets implies supporting nearby makers, utilizing eco-accommodating bundling, and settling on cognizant decisions that limit waste and damage to the climate.

As you set out on this experience, I urge you to embrace the soul of investigation. Find the excellence of lavender's quieting properties, the sustenance of coconut oil, the empowering newness of citrus, and the mitigating impacts of chamomile. Permit nature's miracles to direct you on an excursion of self-disclosure, taking care of oneself, and a more profound association with your general surroundings.

In the sections that follow, you will track down a variety of Do-It-Yourself normal excellence recipes, from facial veils and body scours to hair medicines and sweet-smelling shower mixes. With every creation, you will reveal the genuine embodiment of magnificence - a congruity among inward and external prosperity.

Thus, let this acquaintance be a greeting with step into a universe of healthy magnificence, where nature's gifts become the structure blocks of your taking care of oneself ceremonies. Embrace this excursion with an open heart and an inquisitive soul, and may it lead you to a recently discovered appreciation for the extraordinary force of Do-It-Yourself regular magnificence items.

Hina Victor

Chapter 1

Nourishing Honey and Oatmeal Face Mask

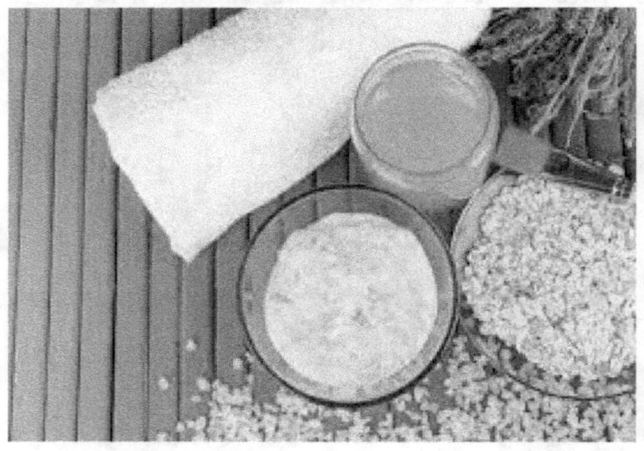

Chasing solid, brilliant skin, there's compelling reason need to look farther than your kitchen storage room. Part 1 acquaints you with the Feeding Honey and Cereal Facial covering, a superb creation that saddles the recuperating powers of two humble yet strong fixings - honey and oats. This regular facial covering is intended to spoil your skin with a feeding mix of nutrients, minerals, and cell reinforcements, leaving you with a delicate, gleaming coloring.

Area 1: The Advantages of Honey for Your Skin

Honey has been venerated for quite a long time for its momentous recuperating properties, making it a dearest fixing in different excellence customs. This part digs into the science behind honey's skin benefits. As a characteristic humectant, honey attracts dampness to your skin, giving profound hydration and forestalling dryness. Its antibacterial and calming properties help in alleviating skin inflammation inclined skin and diminishing redness.

Furthermore, honey's cell reinforcements battle free extremists, advancing an energetic and brilliant tone.

Segment 2: Oats - A Delicate Exfoliate and Soother

Oats, a morning meal staple, serves as a delicate yet compelling exfoliate for your skin. This segment investigates the mitigating and calming properties of oats, which make it reasonable for even the most delicate skin types. Ground cereal goes about as a gentle exfoliate, eliminating dead skin cells and unclogging pores, while its saturating properties leave your skin feeling delicate and graceful.

Area 3: Creating the Sustaining Facial covering

Bit by bit, this segment guides you through the method involved with making the Sustaining Honey and Cereal Facial covering. From choosing the best honey to picking the right sort of cereal, every fixing's significance is featured. You'll find how to join these components into a smooth, lavish cover that is not difficult to apply and delicate on your skin.

Area 4: Applying and Utilizing the Facial covering

When your Feeding Honey and Cereal Facial covering is prepared, this segment gives point by point guidelines on the most proficient method to apply it really. You'll become familiar with the accepted procedures for purging your skin before application, guaranteeing ideal retention of the cover's supplements. With simple to-follow tips, you'll boost the cover's advantages and make a quieting, spa-like involvement with home.

Segment 5: The Aftercare and Skincare Schedule

In the wake of getting your skin this supporting cover, legitimate aftercare is fundamental. This segment presents a basic, regular skincare routine to supplement the advantages of the Supporting Honey and Oats Facial covering. From conditioning to saturating, you'll figure out how to keep up with your brilliant coloring long in the wake of utilizing the cover.

Area 6: Tweaking the Cover for Your Skin Type

Everybody's skin is extraordinary, and this segment offers direction on modifying the facial covering to suit your particular skin type and concerns. Whether you have sleek, dry, mix, or delicate skin, you'll find how to change the fixings to take care of your skin's necessities.

End:

Part 1 finishes up with a sign of the immortal insight of regular excellence cures. The Supporting Honey and Oats Facial covering represents the enchanted that exists in basic, promptly accessible fixings. As you leave on this excursion of making regular excellence items, recollect that the way to brilliant skin is embracing nature's gifts and treating yourself with affection and care.

Chapter 2
Energizing Citrus Body Scrub

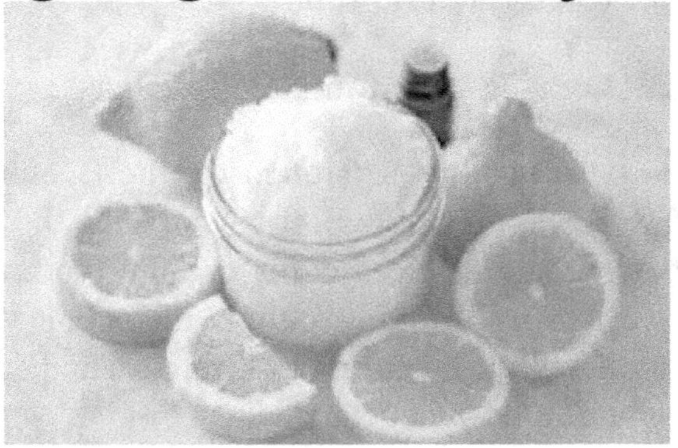

In this part, we dive into the fortifying universe of the Empowering Citrus Body Scour - a great creation that stirs your faculties and rejuvenates your skin. Outfitting the lively and elevating quintessence of citrus organic products, this normal body scour offers a restoring experience that leaves your skin shining with recently discovered energy.

Segment 1: The Energetic Force of Citrus Natural products

Citrus organic products, like oranges, lemons, and grapefruits, are famous for their invigorating smell and high L-ascorbic acid substance. In this segment, we investigate the skincare advantages of citrus organic products, including their capacity to advance collagen creation, light up the skin, and give a stimulating increase in cell reinforcements. Figure out how the normal acids in citrus natural products delicately shed, leaving your skin feeling plush and revived.

Area 2: Choosing the Right Fixings

This part directs you through the method involved with choosing the ideal citrus products of the soil elements for your

Empowering Citrus Body Scour. From picking ready, delicious natural products to consolidating peeling specialists like sugar or salt, you'll figure out how to make a reasonable and compelling scour that suits your skin's necessities.

Segment 3: Creating Your Citrus Body Scour

Bit by bit, we'll walk you through the most common way of creating the Invigorating Citrus Body Scour. Find how to remove the fragrant oils and zing from citrus organic products to imbue your clean with their fortifying pith. With simple to-adhere to directions, you'll make a lively and inspiring clean that leaves your skin feeling empowered and recharged.

Segment 4: The Renewing Experience

Gain proficiency with the prescribed procedures for applying and utilizing the Invigorating Citrus Body Clean. This part offers tips on peeling methods, stressing the significance of delicate round movements to advance blood flow and upgrade the clean's advantages. You'll submerge yourself in a spa-like encounter, changing your washing routine into a reviving and stimulating custom.

Area 5: Post-Scour Skincare Custom

Appropriate post-clean consideration is fundamental to upgrade the advantages of the Invigorating Citrus Body Scour. This part presents a basic yet successful skincare routine to trail behind shedding. From saturating to shielding your skin from the sun, you'll figure out how to keep up with the brilliant sparkle accomplished through the clean.

Segment 6: Customizing Your Citrus Body Scour

Every individual's skin is novel, and in this segment, you'll find how to alter the Empowering Citrus Body Scour to suit your particular necessities and inclinations. Whether you want a seriously shedding surface or an unpretentious fragrance variety, you'll be enabled to fit the scour however you would prefer.

End:

Part 2 closes with a festival of the lively and inspiring characteristics of the Invigorating Citrus Body Clean. By outfitting the dynamic force of citrus organic products, this Do-It-Yourself excellence item offers an actual change as well as a reviving encounter for the brain and soul. Embrace the energy and bliss that citrus brings, and let this clean be a sign of the basic at this point phenomenal marvels nature brings to the table in the domain of regular excellence.

Chapter 3
Glowing Green Tea Toner

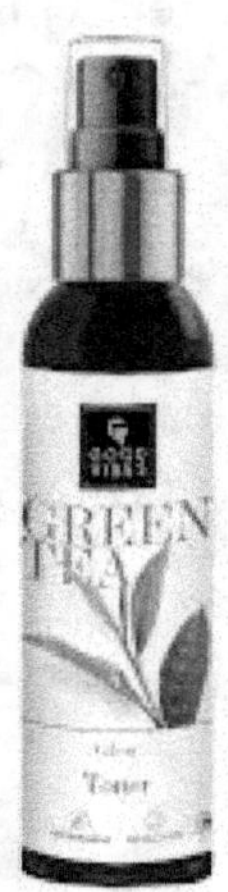

In this section, we drench ourselves in the realm of green tea and its groundbreaking characteristics as we investigate the Shining Green Tea Toner. This regular toner is intended to lift your skincare routine by tackling the strong cancer prevention agents and calming properties of green tea, leaving your skin brilliant and invigorated.

Area 1: The Force of Green Tea for Your Skin

Green tea has been cherished for quite a long time for its various medical advantages, and its skincare benefits are similarly striking. In this segment, we dive into the science behind green tea's skincare ability. As a cell reinforcement force to be reckoned with, green tea assists battle with liberating revolutionaries, limiting untimely maturing and advancing a young composition. Its mitigating properties do some amazing things for relieving and quieting bothered skin, making it appropriate for all skin types.

Area 2: Picking the Right Green Tea

Not all green teas are made equivalent, and this segment guides you in choosing the best assortment for your Gleaming Green Tea Toner. Find out about the various sorts of green tea, for example, matcha, sencha, and black powder, and how each carries its exceptional characteristics to your toner. We likewise talk about the meaning of utilizing natural and top notch green tea leaves to guarantee you receive the greatest rewards for your skin.

Area 3: Supplementing Fixings

To raise the toner's viability, we investigate corresponding fixings that improve green tea's skin-feeding properties. This segment presents a scope of natural concentrates, like chamomile, rosewater, and witch hazel, known for their relieving and conditioning characteristics. Find how these fixings synergize with green tea to make an amicable and fortifying toner.

Area 4: Making the Shining Green Tea Toner

Bit by bit, we guide you through making the Shining Green Tea Toner without any preparation. Gain proficiency with the craft of soaking green tea passes on to extricate their embodiment, and find the various strategies for mixing your toner with natural concentrates. With nitty gritty guidelines, you'll make a rich and reviving toner that will turn into a staple in your skincare schedule.

Segment 5: Application and Integrating the Toner into Your Daily schedule

This part investigates the appropriate use of the Gleaming Green Tea Toner and its mix into your day to day or week by week skincare schedule. You'll get familiar with the best strategies for applying the toner to guarantee ideal assimilation and results. Whether you use it as a conditioning fog or integrate it into your purging routine, this toner will turn into a fundamental stage towards accomplishing a brilliant coloring.

Area 6: Customization for Various Skin Needs

Each individual's skin is extraordinary, and in this segment, we address altering the Sparkling Green Tea Toner to suit explicit skin concerns. Whether you have sleek, dry, delicate, or skin break out inclined skin, you'll find how to adjust the toner's recipe to successfully address your skin's necessities.

End:

Section 3 finishes up with an appreciation for the groundbreaking force of green tea and the Shining Green Tea Toner. With this Do-It-Yourself magnificence item, you embrace the regular excellence ceremonies that honor your skin's wellbeing and prosperity. Permit the cell reinforcements of green tea to sustain and rejuvenate your composition, leaving you with a brilliant shine that mirrors the congruity among nature and taking care of oneself.

Chapter 4

Silky Coconut Milk Hair Conditioner

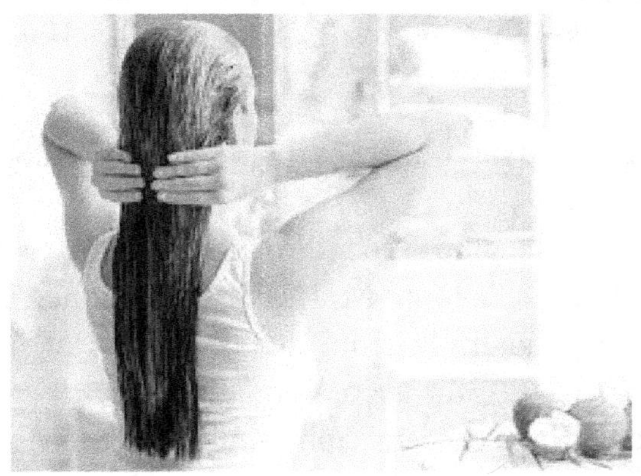

In this section, we adventure into the domain of hair care and present the Plush Coconut Milk Hair Conditioner, a lavish and feeding blend that will change your hair from dreary to tasty. Embracing the regular lavishness of coconut milk, this Do-It-Yourself hair conditioner is intended to hydrate, fortify, and revive your locks, leaving them smooth and brimming with life.

Segment 1: The Miracles of Coconut Milk for Hair

Coconut milk is a gold mine of supplements that have been loved for quite a long time for their extraordinary hair care benefits. In this part, we investigate the science behind coconut milk's benefits for hair wellbeing. Plentiful in fundamental unsaturated fats, proteins, and nutrients E and C, coconut milk profoundly supports and conditions the hair strands, advancing strength and versatility. Its saturating properties battle dryness and frizz, uncovering sparkling, smooth, and reasonable hair.

Area 2: Supplementing Elements for Ideal Outcomes

To improve the advantages of coconut milk, this segment presents corresponding fixings that synergize agreeably with this valuable solution. From the hydrating properties of aloe vera to the reinforcing impacts of honey, we investigate a scope of normal parts that raise the Satiny Coconut Milk Hair Conditioner's viability.

Segment 3: Creating the Extravagant Hair Conditioner

Bit by bit, we guide you through the most common way of making the Satiny Coconut Milk Hair Conditioner. Figure out how to separate coconut milk from new coconuts or utilize excellent canned coconut milk for accommodation. We likewise investigate different detailing choices, obliging different hair types and concerns. With simple to-adhere to guidelines, you'll make a smooth conditioner that vows to change your hair care schedule.

Area 4: Application and Kneading Methods

Appropriate application is vital to receiving the full rewards of the Plush Coconut Milk Hair Conditioner. This part gives experiences into the best strategies for applying the conditioner to your hair, guaranteeing even inclusion and ideal assimilation. You'll find the craft of delicate rubbing to advance course and improve the conditioner's entrance.

Segment 5: Integrating the Conditioner into Your Hair Care Schedule

This segment talks about how to integrate the Plush Coconut Milk Hair Conditioner into your standard hair care schedule. Whether you use it as a week after week profound molding treatment or as a leave-in conditioner for everyday use, this Do-It-Yourself item will change your hair care customs.

Area 6: Customization for Various Hair Types

Each hair type has extraordinary necessities, and in this segment, we investigate how to modify the Sleek Coconut Milk Hair Conditioner to take special care of different hair concerns. From slick and fine hair to wavy and crimped hair, you'll find how to fit the conditioner's recipe to address your particular hair needs.

End:

Part 4 finishes up with a festival of the regular marvels of coconut milk and its capacity to revive and rejuvenate hair. Through the Plush Coconut Milk Hair Conditioner, you embrace a healthy and supporting way to deal with hair care that praises the wellbeing and liveliness of your locks. Permit the lavishness of coconut milk to do something amazing, leaving your hair satiny, smooth, and brilliantly gorgeous, mirroring the excellence of nature's plentiful fortunes.

Chapter 5

Calming Lavender Bath Salts

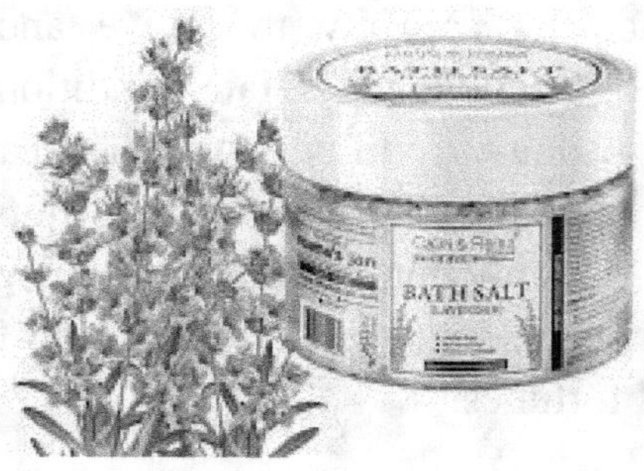

In this part, we welcome you to encounter the encapsulation of unwinding and serenity with Quieting Lavender Shower Salts. Lavender, famous for its alleviating and quieting properties, becomes the overwhelming focus in this wonderful Do-It-Yourself shower item. Drench yourself in an extravagant shower imbued with the pith of lavender, and let go of the burdens of the day as you loosen up in unadulterated joy.

Segment 1: Lavender's Mending Fragrance based treatment

Lavender's helpful properties have been treasured for quite a long time, and in this part, we investigate the science behind its recuperating fragrant healing advantages. Lavender's charming fragrance advances unwinding, diminishes pressure and tension, and helps in prompting serene rest. Find how the smell of lavender functions agreeably with the shower salts to make a peaceful and liberal washing experience.

Segment 2: The Force of Shower Salts for Alleviating the Body

Shower salts are something beyond an extravagance; they offer various advantages for your skin and prosperity. This segment dives into the force of shower salts, for example, Epsom salts and ocean salts, to alleviate tired muscles, diminish aggravation, and detoxify the body. Figure out how these salts work synergistically with lavender to make a quieting and restoring shower custom.

Area 3: Creating Your Quieting Lavender Shower Salts

Bit by bit, we guide you through the method involved with making the Quieting Lavender Shower Salts. From choosing the best lavender rejuvenating balm to picking the ideal mix of shower salts, every fixing assumes a vital part in making a definitive shower salts for unwinding. With simple to-adhere to guidelines, you'll make an extravagant mix that brings the spa experience squarely into the solace of your home.

Segment 4: Upgrading the Shower Insight

This segment gives tips on the most proficient method to improve your shower insight to expand the advantages of the Quieting Lavender Shower Salts. From setting the state of mind with relieving music and faint lighting to consolidating delicate stretches or reflection, you'll figure out how to make a comprehensive washing custom that feeds both body and soul.

Area 5: Skincare After the Shower

Appropriate after-shower care is fundamental for secure in the advantages of the shower salts and lavender. In this segment, we investigate a straightforward and viable skincare routine to trail behind your quiet shower. Figure out how to saturate and spoil your skin, leaving it delicate, flexible, and carefully scented with the quieting aroma of lavender.

Segment 6: Customizing Your Shower Salts

Each individual's inclinations are novel, and this part tends to how to customize the Quieting Lavender Shower Salts to suit your particular preferences. Whether you want a more grounded lavender fragrance or wish to add dried lavender buds for an additional bit of extravagance, you'll be engaged to make a shower salt mix that impacts you.

End:

Part 5 finishes up with a festival of the happy and tranquil experience presented by the Quieting Lavender Shower Salts. Embrace the mending properties of lavender and shower salts as you submerge yourself in a safe house of unwinding and taking care of oneself. Permit the pressure and strain to dissolve away in the alleviating waters, and rise up out of the shower feeling revived, adjusted, and prepared to embrace life's excursion with restored quietness.

Chapter 6
Revitalizing Coffee Eye Cream

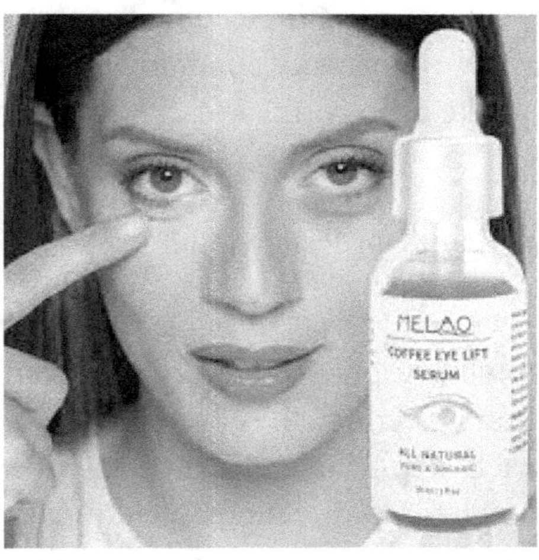

In this section, we plunge into the universe of reviving skincare with the Renewing Espresso Eye Cream - a strong Do-It-Yourself excellence item that makes all the difference for the sensitive skin around your eyes. Tackling the force of espresso and other sustaining fixings, this eye cream is intended to decrease puffiness, reduce dark circles, and revive tired-looking eyes, leaving you looking invigorated and energetic.

Area 1: Espresso's Magnificence Advantages for the Eyes

Espresso is something beyond a morning shot in the arm; it offers a scope of advantages for the skin, particularly around the eyes. In this segment, we investigate the science behind espresso's magnificence benefits for the eyes. The caffeine in espresso functions as a vasoconstrictor, lessening enlarging and puffiness, while its cell reinforcement properties assist with combatting free extremists and diminish indications of maturing. Figure out how espresso's strengthening characteristics make it a strong partner in your eye care schedule.

Area 2: Integral Elements for Eye Restoration

To improve the renewing impacts of espresso, this part presents a choice of integral fixings that work synergistically to revive the eye region. From the feeding properties of almond oil to the skin-lighting up impacts of vitamin E, find how these fixings consolidate to make a powerful eye cream that objectives various eye concerns.

Area 3: Creating Your Renewing Espresso Eye Cream

Bit by bit, we guide you through the most common way of making the Reviving Espresso Eye Cream. From choosing the best coffee beans to injecting the eye cream with advantageous concentrates, each step is intended to boost the cream's viability. With simple to-adhere to directions, you'll make a sumptuous and restoring eye cream that turns into a fundamental piece of your skincare schedule.

Area 4: Application Methods for Ideal Outcomes

This segment offers bits of knowledge into the best procedures for applying the Rejuvenating Espresso Eye Cream to accomplish the best outcomes. You'll learn delicate tapping and kneading methods to further develop blood course and aid the cream's ingestion. Embrace the spoiling custom of applying the eye cream, and experience the loosening up sensation it brings to your day to day daily practice.

Segment 5: Integrating the Eye Cream into Your Skincare Routine

Figure out how to consistently integrate the Reviving Espresso Eye Cream into your day to day or daily skincare routine. Whether utilized as a feature of your morning schedule to battle puffiness or as a calming evening therapy to decrease indications of weakness, this eye cream will turn into a priority item for your magnificence munititions stockpile.

Area 6: Altering for Your Eye Concerns

Every individual's eye concerns are exceptional, and in this segment, we address redoing the Rejuvenating Espresso Eye Cream to suit explicit requirements. Whether you battle with puffiness, dark circles, or scarce differences, you'll find how to adjust the eye cream's recipe to focus on your particular eye concerns really.

End:

Part 6 closes with a festival of the groundbreaking force of espresso and the Reviving Espresso Eye Cream. Through this Do-It-Yourself excellence item, you embrace the magnificence of taking care of oneself and regard for the fragile eye region. Permit the reviving properties of espresso and other feeding fixings to stir and restore your eyes, leaving you with a brilliant and invigorated look that mirrors the dynamic quality of your spirit.

Chapter 7
Moisturizing Aloe Vera Body Lotion

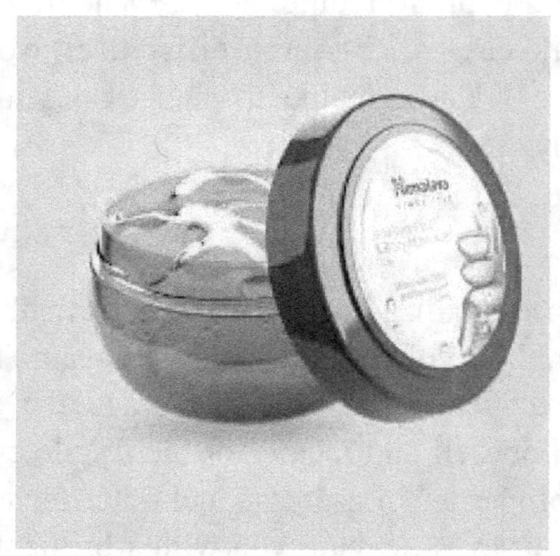

In this section, we jump into the universe of hydrating and sustaining skincare with the Saturating Aloe Vera Body Salve. Aloe vera, known for its alleviating and saturating properties, becomes the overwhelming focus in this sumptuous Do-It-Yourself body salve. Experience a definitive hydration as you embrace the normal integrity of aloe vera, leaving your skin delicate, graceful, and sparkling with imperativeness.

Segment 1: Aloe Vera's Skin-Calming Sorcery

Aloe vera has been respected for quite a long time for its recuperating and mitigating properties, making it a dearest fixing in different skincare items. In this segment, we investigate the science behind aloe vera's skin-alleviating wizardry. Plentiful in nutrients, minerals, and amino acids, aloe vera profoundly hydrates and feeds the skin, advancing a sound and brilliant composition. Find how this flexible plant functions its marvels to change your body salve into a restoring treat for your skin.

Area 2: Reciprocal Elements for Extreme Dampness

To improve the saturating impacts of aloe vera, this part presents correlative fixings that work amicably to secure in dampness and lift skin hydration. From the emollient properties of shea margarine to the skin-mitigating characteristics of chamomile, we investigate a scope of normal parts that hoist the Saturating Aloe Vera Body Moisturizer's viability.

Area 3: Creating Your Hydrating Body Moisturizer

Bit by bit, we guide you through the method involved with making the Saturating Aloe Vera Body Moisturizer. From choosing the freshest aloe vera gel to picking the ideal mix of sustaining oils, every fixing assumes an essential part in making a sleek body cream that extinguishes your skin's thirst. With simple to-adhere to guidelines, you'll make a rich body cream that hoists your day to day taking care of oneself daily practice.

Area 4: Application and Back rub Procedures

This segment gives experiences into the best strategies for applying the Saturating Aloe Vera Body Salve to accomplish greatest hydration and ingestion. Figure out how to spoil your skin with delicate rubbing, advancing dissemination and unwinding. Embrace the sustaining custom of applying the body salve, and experience the luxurious hug it offers your skin.

Area 5: Integrating the Moisturizer into Your Skincare Custom

Figure out how to consistently integrate the Saturating Aloe Vera Body Moisturizer into your everyday skincare routine. Whether utilized as a post-shower treat or as a mitigating cure after sun openness, this body moisturizer will turn into a fundamental piece of your taking care of oneself everyday practice, embracing your skin with affection and sustenance.

Area 6: Customization for Various Skin Types

Each individual's skin is one of a kind, and in this segment, we address modifying the Saturating Aloe Vera Body Cream to suit explicit skin needs. Whether you have dry, delicate, or blend skin, you'll find how to adjust the body salve's recipe to take special care of your skin's novel prerequisites.

End:

Part 7 closes with a festival of the sustaining force of aloe vera and the Saturating Aloe Vera Body Salve. Through this Do-It-Yourself excellence item, you embrace the specialty of taking care of oneself and the magnificence of normal fixings. Permit the mending properties of aloe vera and other skin-supporting fixings to embrace your skin with adoration and hydration, leaving you with a brilliant gleam that mirrors the substance of genuine excellence - a concordance among nature and self.

Chapter 8
Balancing Rosemary and Witch Hazel Toner

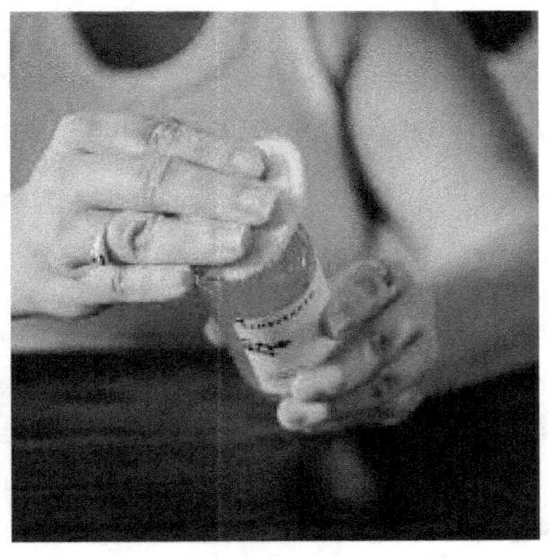

In this section, we investigate the universe of toners and present the Adjusting Rosemary and Witch Hazel Toner - an amicable mix that makes all the difference for your skin's equilibrium and imperativeness. With the intense characteristics of rosemary and witch hazel, this Do-It-Yourself toner is intended to tone, explain, and revive your skin, leaving it invigorated and adjusted.

Segment 1: The Force of Rosemary for Skin Equilibrium

Rosemary has a rich history as a spice known for its therapeutic and skincare properties. In this segment, we investigate the force of rosemary for skin balance. Its astringent properties assist with fixing pores and manage sebum creation, making it an optimal element for those with sleek or skin break out inclined skin. Moreover, rosemary's antibacterial and calming characteristics add to a reasonable and rejuvenated composition.

Segment 2: Witch Hazel's Explaining Enchantment

Witch hazel, a natural concentrate got from the witch hazel bush, is a respected skincare element for its explaining and conditioning benefits. This part digs into the science behind witch hazel's explaining wizardry. Its normal astringent properties assist with refining pores, diminish aggravation, and mitigate disturbed skin. Witch hazel is an incredible expansion to this toner, supplementing rosemary's adjusting characteristics.

Segment 3: Making Your Adjusting Toner

Bit by bit, we guide you through the most common way of making the Adjusting Rosemary and Witch Hazel Toner. From picking the freshest rosemary branches to choosing an excellent witch hazel concentrate, every fixing is chosen to expand the toner's viability. With simple to-adhere to guidelines, you'll make a reviving and empowering toner that raises your skincare schedule.

Area 4: Application Procedures for Ideal Equilibrium

This segment gives experiences into the best strategies for applying the Adjusting Rosemary and Witch Hazel Toner to accomplish the best outcomes. Figure out how to utilize the toner to tone, explain, and balance your skin, advancing an even and brilliant composition. Embrace the invigorating custom of applying the toner, and experience the rejuvenating sensation it brings to your skincare schedule.

Area 5: Integrating the Toner into Your Skincare Routine

Figure out how to flawlessly integrate the Adjusting Rosemary and Witch Hazel Toner into your everyday skincare routine. Whether utilized as a preparing step prior to saturating or as a reviving fog over the course of the day, this toner will turn into a fundamental piece of your excellence weapons store, adding to the ideal wellbeing and equilibrium of your skin.

Area 6: Customization for Various Skin Concerns

Each individual's skin concerns are novel, and in this part, we address redoing the Adjusting Rosemary and Witch Hazel Toner to suit explicit necessities. Whether you have slick, mix, or delicate skin, you'll find how to adjust the toner's equation to really focus on your skin's one of a kind necessities.

End:

Part 8 finishes up with a festival of the amicable mix of rosemary and witch hazel in the Adjusting Rosemary and Witch Hazel Toner. Through this Do-It-Yourself excellence item, you embrace the craft of skincare and the magnificence of normal fixings. Permit the adjusting properties of rosemary and witch hazel to rejuvenate and fit your skin, leaving you with an invigorated and adjusted coloring that mirrors the pith of normal magnificence.

Chapter 9
Hydrating Avocado Hair Mask

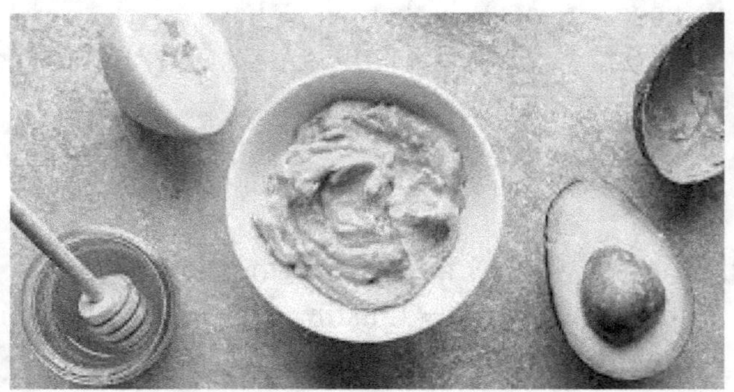

In this part, we set out on an excursion of hair sustenance and present the Hydrating Avocado Hair Veil - a rich Do-It-Yourself treatment that restores and revives your locks. Tackling the rich integrity of avocados, this hair cover is intended to profoundly hydrate, sustain, and reestablish the regular sparkle and imperativeness of your hair.

Segment 1: Avocado's Hair-Supporting Properties

Avocado is a genuine superfood for your hair, loaded with fundamental nutrients, minerals, and unsaturated fats. In this segment, we investigate the hair-feeding properties of avocados. Its high happy of monounsaturated fats and cancer prevention agents helps fix and fortify harmed hair, while its normal oils give extreme dampness and battle dryness. Find how avocados do something amazing to change your hair from dull to astonishing.

Segment 2: Integral Elements for Hair Wellbeing

To improve the hydrating impacts of avocados, this part presents corresponding fixings that work as one to reestablish and keep up with sound hair. From the protein-rich properties of yogurt to the saturating advantages of honey, we investigate a scope of regular parts that raise the Hydrating Avocado Hair Cover's viability.

Area 3: Creating Your Extravagant Hair Veil

Bit by bit, we guide you through the method involved with making the Hydrating Avocado Hair Cover. From choosing the ripest avocados to consolidating the ideal mix of sustaining fixings, each step is intended to boost the veil's adequacy. With simple to-adhere to directions, you'll make a luxurious hair cover that turns into a brilliant treat for your hair.

Area 4: Application Strategies for Ideal Hydration

This segment gives bits of knowledge into the best methods for applying the Hydrating Avocado Hair Cover to accomplish most extreme hydration and sustenance. Figure out how to disseminate the veil equitably all through your hair, zeroing in on the finishes and harmed regions. Embrace the liberal custom of applying the hair cover, and experience the reviving sensation it brings to your hair.

Segment 5: Integrating the Cover into Your Hair Care Schedule

Figure out how to flawlessly integrate the Hydrating Avocado Hair Cover into your week by week hair care schedule. Whether utilized as a week after week profound molding treatment or as a renewing cure after openness to natural stressors, this hair cover will turn into a fundamental piece of your hair care custom, reestablishing your hair's wellbeing and brilliance.

Area 6: Customization for Various Hair Types

Each individual's hair type is extraordinary, and in this part, we address altering the Hydrating Avocado Hair Veil to suit explicit hair needs. Whether you have dry, harmed, or fuzzy hair, you'll find how to adjust the hair cover's equation to really take special care of your hair's remarkable necessities.

End:

Section 9 closes with a festival of the hair-feeding force of avocados and the Hydrating Avocado Hair Cover. Through this Do-It-Yourself magnificence item, you embrace the excellence of hair care and the extravagance of regular fixings. Permit the hydrating properties of avocados and other sustaining fixings to reestablish and restore your hair, leaving you with locks that sparkle with wellbeing and essentialness, mirroring the pith of genuine magnificence - the amicability among nature and taking care of oneself.

Chapter 10

Soothing Chamomile Lip Balm

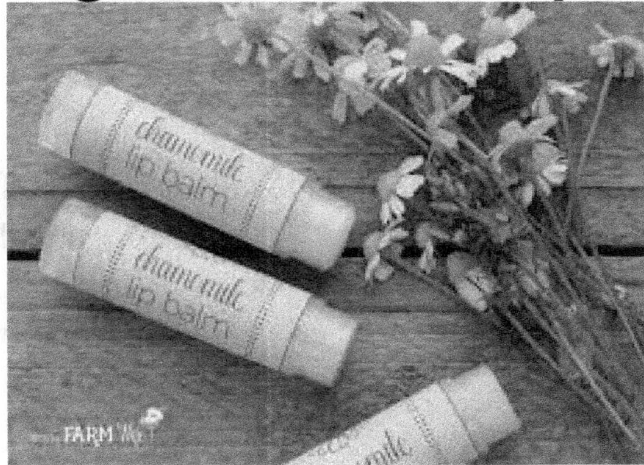

In this last section, we direct our concentration toward the fragile skin of the lips and present the Mitigating Chamomile Lip Emollient - a delicate and feeding Do-It-Yourself lip treatment. Improved with the quieting properties of chamomile, this lip salve is intended to relieve, saturate, and safeguard your lips, leaving them delicate, flexible, and joyfully agreeable.

Area 1: Chamomile's Mending Advantages for the Lips

Chamomile is prestigious for its mending and mitigating properties, making it an ideal element for lip care. In this segment, we investigate the science behind chamomile's advantages for the lips. Its calming and against aggravation properties assist with relieving dry and dried out lips, while its cell reinforcements advance skin fix and restoration. Find how chamomile functions its miracles to change your lips into a kissably delicate and supported mope.

Segment 2: Integral Elements for Lip Sustenance

To improve the alleviating impacts of chamomile, this part presents reciprocal fixings that work couple to give ideal sustenance to your lips. From the hydrating properties of beeswax to the mending advantages of coconut oil, we investigate a scope of regular parts that hoist the Relieving Chamomile Lip Demulcent's viability.

Area 3: Making Your Sumptuous Lip Salve

Bit by bit, we guide you through the method involved with making the Mitigating Chamomile Lip Analgesic. From choosing the best chamomile blossoms to consolidating the ideal mix of lip-adoring fixings, each step is intended to amplify the lip salve's viability. With simple to-adhere to guidelines, you'll make a delectable lip emollient that turns into a spoiling treat for your lips.

Area 4: Application Methods for Ideal Lip Care

This segment gives experiences into the best procedures for applying the Relieving Chamomile Lip Demulcent to accomplish most extreme sustenance and assurance. Figure out how to apply the lip medicine uniformly and liberally, making a calming obstruction that seals in dampness. Embrace the quieting custom of applying the lip demulcent, and experience the solace it brings to your lips.

Area 5: Integrating the Lip Medicine into Your Lip Care Schedule

Figure out how to consistently integrate the Calming Chamomile Lip Analgesic into your day to day lip care schedule. Whether utilized as a day to day saturating treatment or as a short-term lip veil, this lip emollient will turn into a fundamental piece of your lip care custom, guaranteeing your lips are dependably kissably delicate and very much secured.

Area 6: Customization for Individual Lip Care Needs

Each individual's lip care needs are extraordinary, and in this part, we address redoing the Mitigating Chamomile Lip Salve to suit explicit worries. Whether you have dry, delicate, or sun-harmed lips, you'll find how to adjust the lip medicine's equation to actually address your lips' particular necessities.

End:

Part 10 finishes up with a festival of the mending force of chamomile and the Relieving Chamomile Lip Medicine. Through this Do-It-Yourself excellence item, you embrace the magnificence of lip care and the wizardry of regular fixings. Permit the mitigating properties of chamomile and other feeding fixings to comfort and safeguard your lips, leaving you with a delicate and graceful mope that mirrors the embodiment of genuine excellence - a brilliant grin that radiates from a position of self esteem and care.